IMPROVING KIDNEY HEALTH IN 30 DAYS

Kidney Support in 30 Days,
Rehabilitation Plan for Overall Health

By Robert Redfern

About the Author

Your Personal Health Coach
www.MyGoodHealthClub.com

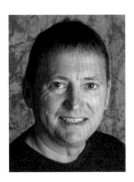

Robert Redfern was born in January 1946. He has helped thousands of people to date in more than 24 countries by providing online health guidance and resources in books, radio interviews, and TV interviews to share his nutritional discoveries. His new book series starts with the Healthier Heart book and is designed to bring all of his health knowledge into one user-friendly format that anyone can understand when pursuing health recovery.

Robert became interested in health when he and his wife Anne began to take charge of their lifestyle in the late 80s. Robert had not paid much attention to his health until 1986, despite Anne's loving influence. It wasn't until Robert's parents Alfred and Marjorie died prematurely in their sixties that he was forced to re-examine his lifestyle choices.

Robert and Anne embraced a new health philosophy as they examined the health community, medical treatments, and common health issues. After researching the root cause of disease, they discovered that diet and lifestyle choices were the two most pivotal factors that contribute to overall health and well-being. Robert and Anne decided to make major changes in their diet and lifestyle, while utilizing **HealthPoint**™ acupressure. The changes that they saw were exceptional.

In addition to improved health, Robert and Anne both look and feel like they have more vitality than they did decades before they started their new health plan. Currently, Robert, 68, and Anne continue to make healthy choices to live energetically and youthfully, based on a foundation of Natural Health.

ROBERT REDFERN: YOUR PERSONAL HEALTH COACH
Provides step-by-step guidance on -

Kidney Disease Prevention and Recovery:

Achieve and Maintain Healthy Kidney Function Through Long-Term Rehabilitation

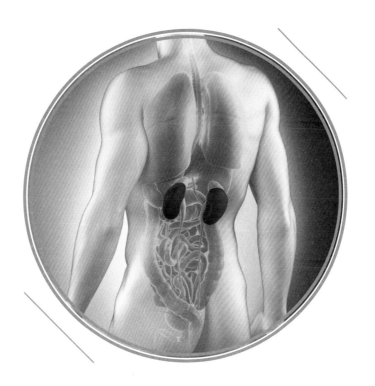

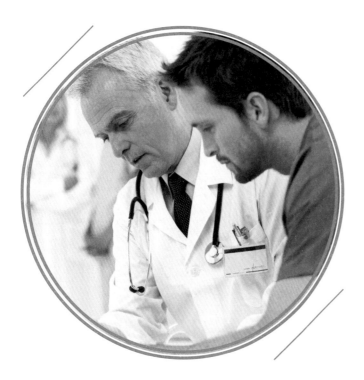

Publisher:

Naturally Healthy Publications. All rights reserved.

Publication printed in the United Kingdom.

Publisher's Note:

This book is not intended to diagnose any disease or offer medical advice. The intention of the book is only to provide information for the reader so that they can make healthy lifestyle choices.

Warning:

Some of the information in this book may contradict advice from your physician; nonetheless, content is based on the science of natural health.

CONTENTS

YOUR COMMITMENT PLAN FOR BETTER KIDNEY HEALTH

TODAY	I DID THIS	SIGNED	DATE
I Committed	To restoring and supporting my health for all of my life.		
I Committed	To drinking 6-8 glasses of water per day with a pinch of sodium bicarbonate in each glass.		
I Committed	To spending time in the sun for 20 minutes each day (except when not advised).		
I Read	Robert's *Improving Kidney Health in 30 Days* Book.		
I Ordered	The recommended supplements to support my plan and healing.		
I Planned	My Daily Menu with **ReallyHealthyFoods.com.**		
I Started	My breathing exercises.		
I Started	Massaging the appropriate acupressure points.		
I Reread	Robert's *Improving Kidney Health in 30 Days* Book.		
I Reviewed	The recommended supplements to support my plan and healing.		
I Reviewed	My water intake.		
I Reviewed	My Daily Menu.		
I Reviewed	My breathing exercises.		
I Reviewed	My life-giving sun exposure (except when not advised).		
I Reviewed	How to massage the appropriate acupressure points.		
I Recommitted	To restoring and supporting my health for all of my life.		
I Recommitted	Robert's *Improving Kidney Health in 30 Days* Book.		
I Recommitted	To the recommended supplements to support my plan and healing.		
I Recommitted	To my water intake.		
I Recommitted	To following my Daily Menu.		
I Recommitted	To doing my breathing exercises.		
I Recommitted	To life-giving sun exposure (except when not advised).		
I Recommitted	To massaging the appropriate acupressure points.		

What Is Kidney Disease?

Kidney disease is considered by many to be the silent killer. It is the ninth leading cause of death in the Western world. More than 20 million adults over the age of 20 have kidney disease—though many don't know they have the condition.

The kidneys are small but mighty. Kidneys are fist-sized organs shaped like beans. Two kidneys can be found in the middle of your back, on the left and right of the spine.

> *Kidneys are essential to the body. They filter out excess water and waste from the blood to make urine.*

Most people are familiar with this basic kidney function, but kidneys do much more:

- **Kidneys control blood pressure, vital to balanced health.**

- **Kidneys produce hormones needed by the body.**

- **Kidneys monitor fluid content, adjust mineral levels, and activate vitamin D, an essential vitamin absorbed from the sun.**

- **Kidneys produce urine to excrete waste and reabsorb water, glucose, and amino acids.**

When kidneys become damaged, waste quickly accumulates in the body. "Renal" is a word commonly associated with kidney health. Kidney function may be referred to as renal function. Your doctor may call kidney failure *renal failure*.

Kidney disease occurs when damaged kidneys can no longer effectively filter blood. Once waste builds up as a result of kidney damage, it can cause a domino effect in the body that ultimately leads to poor health.

Kidney damage is likely to occur over several years and may be diagnosed as chronic kidney disease (CKD). Chronic kidney disease differs from a sudden change in kidney health related to injury, illness, or medication, otherwise known as acute kidney injury.

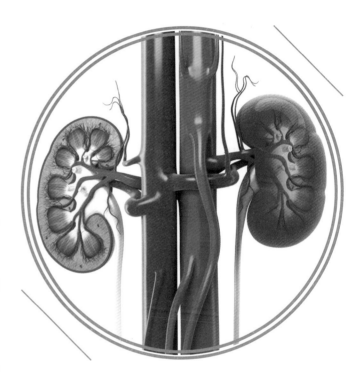

Signs of Chronic Kidney Disease

Chronic kidney disease, or chronic kidney failure, occurs through a gradual loss of renal function. Once this gradual deterioration progresses to an advanced stage, waste, electrolytes, and fluid will build up in the body at dangerous levels.

Early stages of chronic kidney disease are more difficult to detect. As symptoms intensify, chronic kidney disease may be diagnosed when renal function has greatly declined.

It is important to address kidney health if you have been diagnosed with chronic kidney disease. If CKD goes untreated, complications like anemia, weak bones, high blood pressure, poor nutrition, and even nerve damage can result. Chronic kidney disease can increase the risk of heart and blood vessel disease. Long-term chronic kidney disease can lead to kidney failure, requiring dialysis or a kidney transplant to survive. However, CKD patients are more likely to die from heart disease than kidney failure.

Symptoms of chronic kidney disease may include:

- Vomiting/nausea
- Loss of appetite
- Weakness/fatigue
- Difficulty sleeping
- Puffiness around eyes, especially in the morning
- Changes in urine output
- Increased urge to urinate, especially at night
- Difficulty concentrating
- Swollen ankles/feet
- Muscle cramps/twitches
- Chronic itching
- Shortness of breath, related to fluid buildup in the lungs
- Chest pain, related to fluid buildup around heart lining
- Hypertension, or high blood pressure

Early intervention can help to prevent kidney failure.

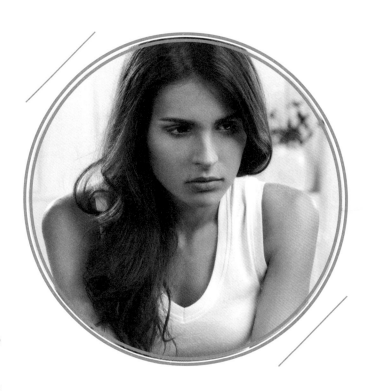

Source: National Kidney Foundation

What Are the Different Types of Kidney Disease?

❧ Kidney disease includes any disorder, condition, or disease that affects the kidneys.

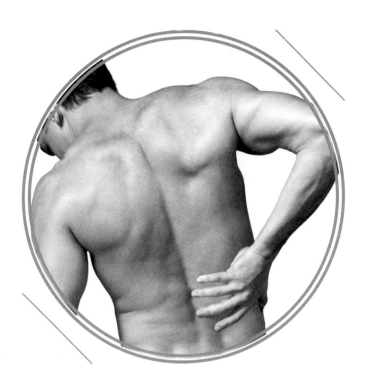

Kidney disease may be broken down into the following categories:

- **Acute Kidney Disease:** Acute kidney disease is characterized by a sudden loss of kidney function triggered by high levels of waste byproducts collected in the blood. Causes may include severe infection, dehydration, injury, kidney stones, or damage from toxins or medication.

- **Chronic Kidney Disease:** Kidney damage occurs gradually over several years until permanent kidney disease develops. Additional treatment may be needed for CKD complications, including anemia and nerve damage.

- **Pediatric Kidney Disease:** Both acute and chronic kidney disease can develop in children. Pediatric kidney disease may be caused by genetic factors, birth defects, infection, systemic diseases, trauma, Nephrotic Syndrome, and urine blockage or reflux. Birth defects and hereditary diseases are the top causes of kidney failure in children under four.

- **Polycystic Kidney Disease:** Polycystic kidney disease (PKD) is the most common inherited kidney disease in Western countries; it affects 12 million people worldwide. Polycystic kidney disease results in the growth of kidney cysts that compromise kidney structure and function. Cysts can spread to other organs, namely the liver. PKD is the third most common cause of kidney failure.

Source: The Rogosin Institute

Kidney disease may also include:

- **Alport Syndrome:** Genetic disorder common in young men that damages the blood vessels of the kidneys; may also cause severe hearing loss.

- **Diabetic Nephropathy:** Kidney damage caused by diabetes and high blood sugar.

- **Fabry Disease:** Rare genetic disorder where fatty deposits accumulate in blood vessels to damage the kidneys, heart, and brain.

- **Focal Segmental Glomerulosclerosis:** Scarring of the small blood vessels in the kidneys (glomeruli).

- **Glomerulonephritis:** Inflammation of the small blood vessels used for filtering in the kidneys.

- **IgA Nephropathy (Berger's Disease):** Buildup of IgA protein in the kidneys that causes blood vessel inflammation.

- **Kidney Stones:** Solid mineral concretions formed in urine in the kidneys; large calcium stones can block urine flow to cause severe pain. Long-term kidney stone obstructions can lead to scarring and kidney damage.

- **Minimal Change Disease:** MCG is the leading cause of Nephrotic Syndrome in children and may be related to NSAID use, tumors, vaccinations, viral infections, and allergic reactions.

- **Nephrotic Syndrome:** Nonspecific disorder characterized by damage to the kidneys' blood vessels, resulting in protein in urine and edema. MCG (Minimal Change Disease) may be used interchangeably with Nephrotic Syndrome.

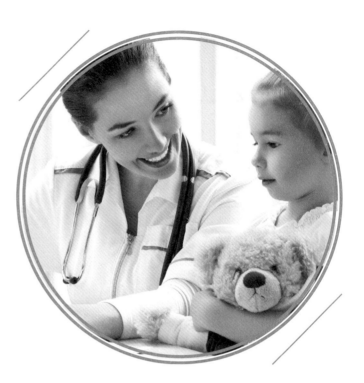

Source: University Kidney Research Organization

What Causes Kidney Disease?

Kidney disease may be caused by:

- Diet high in sugar

- Diet high in starchy carbs

- Overly acidic diet

- Diabetes

- High blood pressure

- Sodium bicarbonate deficiency

- Pharmaceutical drugs

- Immune system conditions, including HIV/AIDS, hepatitis B, hepatitis C, and lupus

- Multiple urinary tract infections that result in scarring

- Inflammation of the kidney's tiny filters (glomeruli)

- Polycystic kidney disease

- Congenital birth defects

New Cases of Kidney Failure by Primary Diagnosis: CDC, 2011

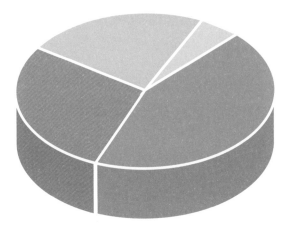

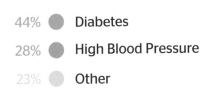

44% ● Diabetes

28% ● High Blood Pressure

23% ● Other

5% ● Unknown

Type 1 and 2 diabetes and high blood pressure are the most common causes of chronic kidney disease.

It is important to understand that type 2 diabetes and high blood pressure are lifestyle conditions. These health issues are caused by eating pastries, bread, cookies, breakfast cereals, pizza, white rice, potatoes, parsnips, pasta, sugary drinks, and other high-sugar foods.

Avoiding unnatural foods and supplementing with missing nutrients can correct serious health issues like diabetes and high blood pressure, in the majority of cases. Addressing these health issues can restore kidney health in the early stages of kidney disease and can help to prevent irreparable kidney damage.

The best way to control kidney disease is by managing blood pressure and blood sugar through a non-inflammatory lifestyle.

Chronic Kidney Disease Risk Factors

Chronic kidney disease risk factors may include:

- Age - over 65

- Genetics

- Ethnicity - American Indian, Asian-American, and African-American

- Smoking

- Obesity

- High cholesterol

- Autoimmune disease

- Type 1 and 2 diabetes

- Cardiovascular disease

- Atherosclerosis

- Kidney or bladder cancer

- Kidney infection

- Liver cirrhosis or failure

High blood pressure and diabetes are the major risk factors for chronic kidney disease that are under your control. One out of three adults with diabetes has chronic kidney disease. One out of five adults with high blood pressure has chronic kidney disease. Incidences of chronic kidney disease increase over the age of 65, and CKD may also run in families.

> *Men with chronic kidney disease are 50% more likely than women to experience kidney failure.*

Chronic kidney disease is becoming a worldwide epidemic related to a rise in hypertension (high blood pressure), diabetes, and cardiovascular disease. CKD rates have increased throughout the developed world, in the United States, Europe, Asia, Australia, and areas of India, China, and Africa.

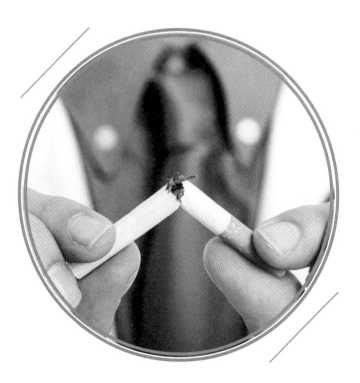

Source: CDC

Sodium Bicarbonate for Chronic Kidney Disease

Researchers believe that sodium bicarbonate, a.k.a. baking soda, can help to slow the progression of chronic kidney disease. Baking soda is a product you're likely to find around the house. It can be used for baking and cleaning, as well as a home remedy for acid indigestion.

Seriously ill patients with chronic kidney disease (CKD) may have to spend hours a day hooked up to a dialysis machine to filter waste and substitute kidney function. Patients in need of dialysis or a kidney transplant may benefit from a simpler and more effective approach: a baking soda supplement for CKD patients with low bicarbonate levels.

Low bicarbonate levels in CKD patients are referred to as metabolic acidosis. Royal London Hospital studied this effect in 134 patients with chronic kidney disease. CKD patients were administered a small daily sodium bicarbonate supplement, in addition to their regular treatment protocol.

One year later, patients who received sodium bicarbonate showed significantly slower kidney function decline compared to patients who did not receive the baking soda supplement. Patients in the sodium bicarbonate group had a rate of kidney decline considered slightly above the normal effects of aging.

> *Even more impressive was the fact that patients who took sodium bicarbonate tablets were less likely to progress into end-stage renal disease and require dialysis.*

Sodium bicarbonate has been used as a chemotherapy and radiation adjunct to protect against kidney damage. Because of its ability to neutralize acid in the blood and urine, sodium bicarbonate has even been used in emergency rooms to provide relief for serious kidney problems and treat some medication overdose.

Since the kidneys are vital to flush excess acid from the diet, a patient with kidney disease is likely to collect acid in the body. Excess acid can change metabolism. Sodium bicarbonate supplementation is recommended by the American Association of Kidney Patients to slow down kidney disease and restore function.

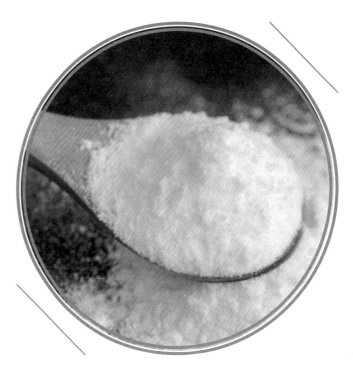

Source: JASN September 1, 2009 vol. 20 no. 9 2075-2084

The Sodium Bicarbonate and Sea Salt Connection

The beauty of sodium bicarbonate as a treatment for kidney disease is that it is an entirely natural substance. Baking soda can be found in soil, in the ocean, in food, and in the body. Baking soda is a neutralizing compound that can be used as a medicinal remedy.

> *Your body makes sodium bicarbonate to act as an acid buffer.*

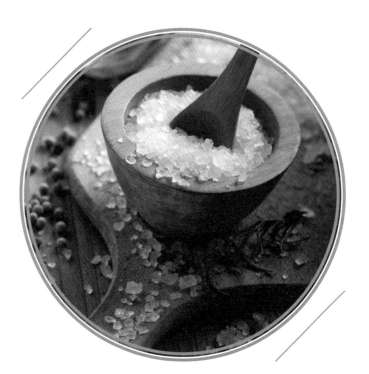

Sodium bicarbonate is being constantly produced by the stomach's cover cells to alkalize acidic foods and liquids that you eat. This sodium bicarbonate produced in the stomach also buffers respiratory and metabolic acids to maintain delicate blood and tissue alkalinity (7.365 pH).

Critical alkaline balance in your body can be compromised by low levels of sodium bicarbonate. Your body may be unable to produce sodium bicarbonate because of a very common mineral salt deficiency in the diet.

According to Robert O. Young, D.Sc., Ph.D., NMD, low sodium bicarbonate levels directly affect the stomach, pancreas, and kidneys. Dr. Thomas P. Kennedy of the American Medical Association confirms that sodium bicarbonate ions can neutralize acids that trigger chronic inflammation; sodium bicarbonate can be beneficial in treating chronic inflammatory and autoimmune diseases. Low sodium bicarbonate levels related to mineral salt deficiency have been directly linked to inflammation, edema, diabetes, cancer, and kidney disease.

Your body needs raw organic salt in the diet to produce sodium bicarbonate. For a completely healthy body, raw sea or rock salt is essential.

> *Anyone worth their salt can tell you that!*

Source: Sodium bicarbonate uses and science by Robert O. Young, D.Sc., Ph.D., NMD

Why It Pays to Be Proactive About Kidney Disease

The American Association of Kidney Patients confirms that 7.5% of patients with moderate chronic kidney disease do not know they have the condition. A growing number of people who have been diagnosed with CKD do very little about it.

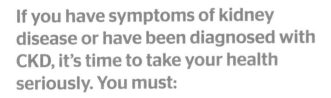

Kidney disease can be treated and managed if it is caught early on.

Making the essential lifestyle changes outlined in this book will pave the way to a healthy, balanced life. You can restore kidney health and greatly reduce symptoms of chronic kidney disease, in many cases. Treating kidney disease early can also help to prevent heart disease.

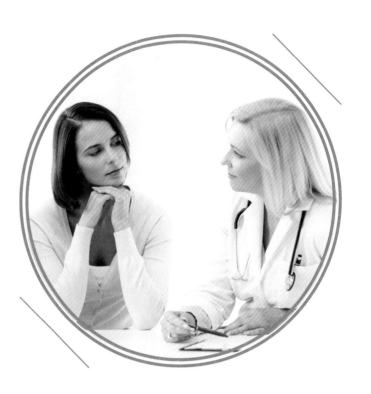

Kidney disease left untreated without lifestyle changes will not go away. It will get worse. Over the long-term, chronic kidney disease will cause kidney failure or even heart failure. Once kidneys fail, a drastic treatment like dialysis or a transplant will be needed to save a life. Long-term kidney disease can lead to a number of health complications that could otherwise be prevented, including heart attack and stroke.

If you have symptoms of kidney disease or have been diagnosed with CKD, it's time to take your health seriously. You must:

1. **Commit to a new, non-inflammatory lifestyle.**
2. **Learn to balance blood pressure.**
3. **Learn to manage or reduce diabetes.**
4. **Increase your antioxidant intake.**
5. **Start bicarbonate therapy right away.**

The Western Un-Natural Food Diet

A diet which will definitely hinder one's recovery from kidney disease is the Western Un-Natural Food Diet.

> Nothing affects us more than what we choose to eat at least three to four times a day, every day.

Most of us lack the essential nutrients in our diet needed for good health, perpetuating inflammation. This absence of nutrients combined with one or several other unhealthy lifestyle choices can perpetuate kidney disease.

The "Balanced Western Diet" (now better described as the Western Un-Natural Food Diet) is the number one disease-promoting and inflammation-producing diet in modern society. It is consumed more and more on a daily basis.

This highly inflammatory diet is made up of sugary foods in the form of breads, pastas, cereals, and potatoes. The Western Un-Natural Food Diet is way too high in unhealthy fats and lacks the antioxidants and phytochemicals that are crucial for eliminating free radicals. This all too common diet is lacking in high-fiber foods and the foods that provide essential nutrients necessary to find relief from kidney disease.

These missing foods include:

- Vegetables
- Dark-skinned fruits
- Nuts
- Seeds
- **Beans (except when temporarily contraindicated for recovery)**

Antioxidants are essential for sufferers of CKD. Research has confirmed that antioxidants can help to slow the development of chronic kidney disease in patients with CKD.

Where can you find vital antioxidants to protect against advanced kidney disease? Antioxidants are best found in a Really Healthy Foods diet full of fresh, whole foods, along with powerful supplements to provide missing nutrients. Antioxidants can relieve whole body inflammation and support the healing process.

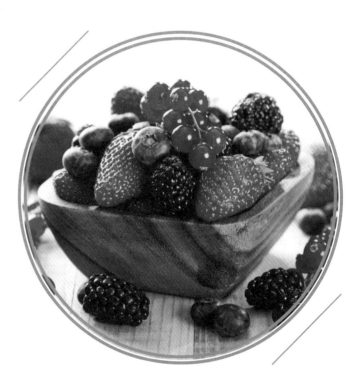

Source: Jun M, Venkataraman V, Razavian M, Cooper B, Zoungas S, Ninomiya T, et al. Antioxidants for chronic kidney disease. Cochrane Database Syst Rev. 2012;10:CD008176.

Can I Reverse Kidney Disease?

I prefer not to use the word "cure" when talking about these health conditions since many cases are directly related or exacerbated by lifestyle factors.

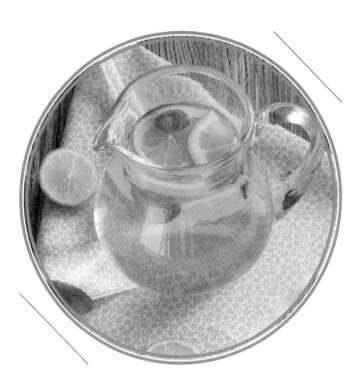

Cure is a popular medical buzzword, although the medical field cannot provide cures. (Many people argue that this is on purpose since it would put Big Pharma out of business.) Every health condition has a cause. When you take away the underlying cause and follow a non-inflammatory lifestyle, your body will have the support it needs to repair itself, in many cases.

When you remove the cause and support your body with healthy lifestyle choices and nutrients, you can often grow healthy again. You may call this a cure, but I believe it to be making healthy lifestyle choices.

Since these health conditions are inflammatory, a non-inflammatory lifestyle is a must. It's important to stay hydrated by drinking six to eight 16 ounce (500 ml) glasses of pure, clean water per day. You can heal your body with vital nutrients and antioxidants found in vitamins, minerals, healthy carbohydrates, amino acids, and essential fatty acids.

Healing starts with nutritional therapy.

Detoxification may be uncomfortable at first, but this too will pass.

Sensible eating can support your recovery.

. . . transform your health with a balanced lifestyle and essential nutrients. . .

Essential Nutrients

According to research, these nutrients can manage or prevent kidney disease in most cases:

Sodium Thiocyanate and Sodium Hypothiocyanate - Clear any remaining infection in the cells.

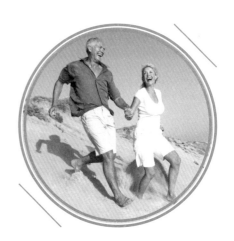

Nascent Iodine - Essential for a completely healthy body; aids the body in processes, such as detoxification, protecting cells and tissues, increasing metabolism, and improving energy.

Serrapeptase, Nattokinase, Protease, and Lipase - Serrapeptase gives powerful support to the digestive system and lowers inflammation.

Curcumin – Provides superior support and pain relief for digestive problems, the liver, and the gallbladder.

29 Super Strain Probiotic – Contains a proprietary blend of Leonardite and 29 probiotic microflora "Soil Based Organisms" (SBOs) to support the digestive tract.

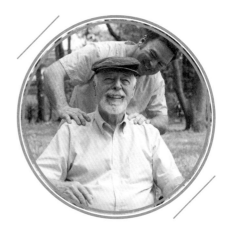

Vitamin B1, B2, B3, B5, B6, and B12, et al. - Supports healthy homocysteine levels, giving a healthy boost to the immune system and improving B12 absorption.

Vitamin C, D3, ExSelen (Selenium), Zinc, Elderberry Fruit Extract 4:1, et al. - Protects against infection and maintains a balanced immune system.

Cinnamon Bark, Cedar Leaves, Wild Rose Root, Fenugreek Seed, Damiana Leaf, et al. - Powerful herbal formula designed to cleanse and support kidney health.

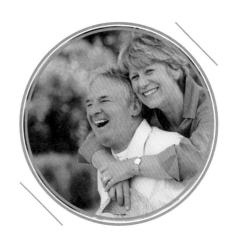

4. Why Doesn't My Doctor Tell Me I Can Get Better?

You can use the Kidney Rehabilitation Program to improve your health! Your doctor has an obligation to stick with the prescription drug outline that fits into the pharmaceutical industry monopoly. This includes the AMA in the US and the GMC in the UK.

Make no mistake - these organizations make money off basic healthcare for sick individuals. They don't have a business model that promotes actual health recovery in any way, shape, or form. These organizations push a patented prescription drug protocol that allows them to charge outrageous prices for drug use over a lifetime. At the very best, these drugs may help the patient to feel better, but in many scenarios, they could lead to their death.

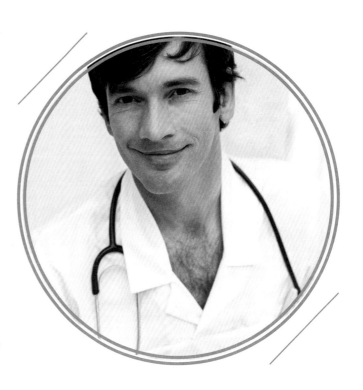

> *These industries won't support long-term health recovery in any circumstance!*

These organizations are protected by the FDA in the US and the MHRA in the UK. They receive backing from powerful political parties that continue to fund the disease-promoting monopoly I have just described.

Yet when you follow the Kidney Rehabilitation Program to the letter, you can see results within 30 days.

Your Kidney Rehabilitation Plan
10 Steps for Long-Term Health Recovery

This self-recovery protocol can be used by sufferers of kidney disease, in most cases:

1 Clear inflammation and facilitate healing.

2 Supplement missing nutrients.

3 Boost your immune system.

4 Drink more water.

5 Cut out unnatural foods.

6 Eat really healthy foods.

7 Stay active daily.

8 Learn proper breathing.

9 Stimulate acupressure points.

10 Get more sun exposure.

It's almost impossible not to see significant health changes after applying many of the points in this 10 Step Plan. You can clear up numerous symptoms and may see a full recovery, in many cases.

For details of the suggested plans, turn to **page 32**.

1. Clear Inflammation and Facilitate Healing.
Basic Plan

- **Nascent Iodine** - Take 5 drops, 3 times per day in 20ml of water, swish around the mouth for 30 seconds before swallowing. Build over 2 weeks to 15 x 3 until well and then slowly reduce back to 5 x 3. Take 1st dose on waking, 2nd mid-morning, and 3rd mid-afternoon. Iodine is essential for a completely healthy body. Note that Iodine needs a supplement containing Selenium to activate it, such as Active Life, D.I.P. Daily Immune Protection, or B4 Health Spray.

- **BlockBuster AllClear** -Take 2 capsules, 3 times per day, 30 minutes before eating a meal with water; reduce to 1 x 3 after a month. BlockBuster AllClear contains Serrapeptase, Nattokinase, Protease, and Lipase. Serrapeptase gives powerful support for the digestive system and lowers inflammation.

- **Curcuminx4000** - Take 1 capsule, 3 times per day with BlockBuster. Curcumin provides superior support and pain relief for digestive problems, the liver, and the gallbladder.

2. Supplement Missing Nutrients.
Advanced Plan

- **Nascent Iodine** - Take 5 drops, 3 times per day in 20ml of water, swish around the mouth for 30 seconds before swallowing. Build over 2 weeks to 15 x 3 until well and then slowly reduce back to 5 x 3. Take 1st dose on waking, 2nd mid-morning, and 3rd mid-afternoon. Iodine is essential for a completely healthy body. Note that Iodine needs a supplement containing Selenium to activate it, such as Active Life, D.I.P. Daily Immune Protection, or B4 Health Spray.

- **BlockBuster AllClear** -Take 2 capsules, 3 times per day, 30 minutes before eating a meal with water; reduce to 1 x 3 after a month. BlockBuster AllClear contains Serrapeptase, Nattokinase, Protease, and Lipase. Serrapeptase gives powerful support for the digestive system and lowers inflammation.

- **Curcuminx4000** - Take 1 capsule, 3 times per day with BlockBuster. Curcumin provides superior support and pain relief for digestive problems, the liver, and the gallbladder.

- **Prescript-Assist - 29 Super Strain Probiotic** - Take 1 capsule, 2 times a day (can be opened and mixed with food) and then for maintenance at the rate of 1 every 3 days. This is the next-generation, clinically-proven vegan probiotic supplement.

- **B4 Health Spray** - Take 6 sprays daily. Supports healthy homocysteine levels, gives a healthy boost to the immune system, and improves the absorption of B12.

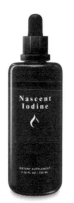
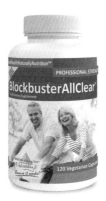
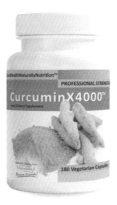

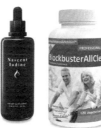
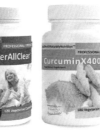
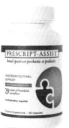
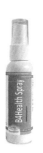

Please note that recommended products and prices may vary and be subject to change, depending on stock level and manufacturer availability.

21

3. Boost Your Immune System.
Ultimate Plan

- **Nascent Iodine** - Take 5 drops, 3 times per day in 20ml of water, swish around the mouth for 30 seconds before swallowing. Build over 2 weeks to 15 x 3 until well and then slowly reduce back to 5 x 3. Take 1st dose on waking, 2nd mid-morning, and 3rd mid-afternoon. Iodine is essential for a completely healthy body. Note that Iodine needs a supplement containing Selenium to activate it, such as Active Life, D.I.P. Daily Immune Protection, or B4 Health Spray.

- **BlockBuster AllClear** -Take 2 capsules, 3 times per day, 30 minutes before eating a meal with water; reduce to 1 x 3 after a month. BlockBuster AllClear contains Serrapeptase, Nattokinase, Protease, and Lipase. Serrapeptase gives powerful support for the digestive system and lowers inflammation.

- **Curcuminx4000** - Take 1 capsule, 3 times per day with BlockBuster. Curcumin provides superior support and pain relief for digestive problems, the liver, and the gallbladder.

- **Prescript-Assist - 29 Super Strain Probiotic** - Take 1 capsule, 2 times a day (can be opened and mixed with food) and then for maintenance at the rate of 1 every 3 days. This is the next-generation, clinically-proven vegan probiotic supplement.

- **B4 Health Spray** - Take 6 sprays daily. Supports healthy homocysteine levels, gives a healthy boost to the immune system, and improves the absorption of B12.

- **D.I.P. Daily Immune Protection** - Take 1 capsule, twice daily with food. Protects against infection and maintains a balanced immune system.

- **Kidney Rescue** - Take 2-5 tablets, 5 times per day, 6 days per week. Kidney Rescue cleanses the liver, while providing adrenal support.

ALSO, TAKE:

- 6-8 glasses of water per day with a pinch of bicarbonate of soda in each glass.

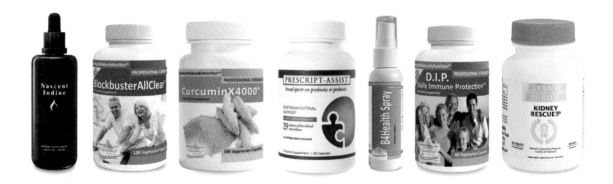

Optional - But Highly Recommended for At Least 1 to 2 Months

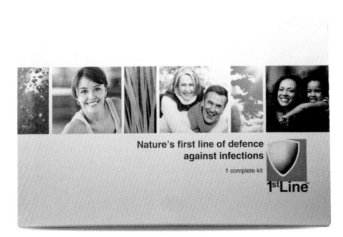

1st Line (Thiocyanate) Immune Support Kit - Take 1 kit daily for 3 days (total of 3). 1st Line should always be taken at least 90 minutes before and after food, approximately. 3 kits are the minimum, and in serious conditions, 10 kits over 10 days are better if finances allow. This kit clears any infection remaining in the cells.

4. Drink More Water.

Drink at least 6-8 glasses of RO filtered or distilled water each day; add a generous pinch of baking soda to each glass. This step is essential for patients with chronic kidney disease.

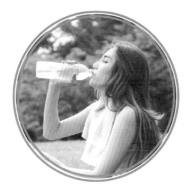

5. Cut Out Unnatural Foods.

Until you've achieved full recovery, cut out starchy carbohydrates altogether, i.e. pastries, cookies, breads, breakfast cereals, pasta, and potatoes, as well as processed foods and milk products.

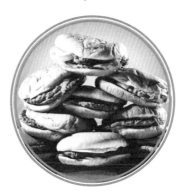

Note: Don't eat turnips, parsnips, and rice, except for small portions of wild rice, brown rice, and sweet potatoes/yams.

6. Eat Really Healthy Foods.

Make sure to eat some of these foods every two hours for the first few months of recovery:

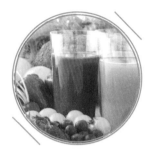

Eat 9-14 servings of fresh or frozen vegetables each day: try them in soups, steamed, stir-fried, juiced, etc. Eat 50% raw, juiced vegetables (preferably organic) and use the pulp to make soup. Blended veggies promote easier digestion.

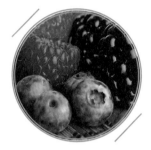

Eat 5 servings of dark-skinned fruits (like cherries, red grapes, blueberries, etc.) that are rich in antioxidants each day.

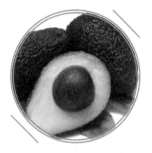

Remember that avocados are a number one superfood with almost a complete spectrum of nutrients. If they are readily available in your area, try to eat at least two a day to promote health recovery. Avocados support CKD, heart disease, diabetes, and even cancer recovery.

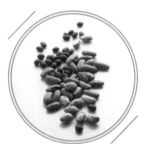

Eat 5 servings of nuts, beans, and seeds (soaked, mashed nuts and seeds).

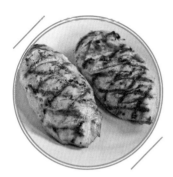

Eat pasture-fed chicken and other meats, only a few servings per week. Grass-fed meat is recommended above corn or grain-fed meat sources.

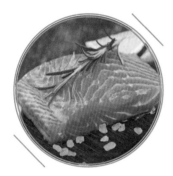

Eat a minimum of 3-4 servings of oily fish each week, if you eat fish. Choose a variety of healthy fish like mackerel, sardines, salmon, etc. Canned fish is a nutritious option, although wild caught fish is recommended.

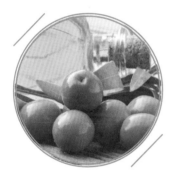

Add healthy oils to your favorite foods, like krill, omega 3, hemp, coconut, and olive oils. Pair with healthy carbohydrate alternatives, like amaranth, quinoa, buckwheat, and chai and millet seeds. You can also try couscous, if you aren't allergic to gluten protein (celiac disease).

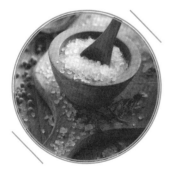

Add 3-5 teaspoons of sea or rock salt, depending on the heat and your body mass, to water or food each day. Remember that sea or rock salt does not contain the important mineral iodine, so Nascent Iodine is recommended in your Rehabilitation Plan.

Recommended Vegetables

Note: Vegetables may not be available in all countries.

- Artichoke
- Asian Vegetable Sprouts (Wheat, Barley, Alfalfa, etc.)
- Asparagus
- Avocado
- Beetroot
- Broad Beans
- Broccoli
- Brussel Sprouts
- Cabbage (various types)
- Capsicum
- Carrots
- Cauliflower
- Celeriac
- Choko
- Cucumber
- Dandelion Leaves
- Dried Peas
- Eggplant (Aubergine)
- Fennel
- Garden Peas
- Garlic
- Kale
- Kohlrabi
- Kumara
- Lettuce (Kos and various types)
- Mangetout Peas
- Mushrooms
- Okra
- Onions (Red and White)
- Petit Pois Peas
- Radishes
- Runner Beans
- Seaweed - all types (Kelp, Wakame, Noni, etc.)
- Silver Beet
- Spinach
- Squash
- Sugar Snap Peas
- Zucchini (Courgettes)

Recommended Fruits

Note: Fruits may not be available in all countries.

- Apple
- Apricot
- Avocado
- Bilberries
- Blackberries
- Blackcurrants
- Blueberries
- Cherimoya
- Cherries
- Damsons
- Dates
- Durian
- Figs
- Gooseberries
- Grapefruit
- Grapes
- Kiwi fruit
- Limes
- Lychees
- Mango
- Nectarine
- Orange
- Pear
- Pineapple
- Plum/Prune (Dried Plum)
- Pomegranate
- Rambutan
- Raspberries
- Salal berry
- Satsuma
- Strawberries
- Tangerine
- Western raspberry (Blackcap)

The Garden of Eden Pyramid

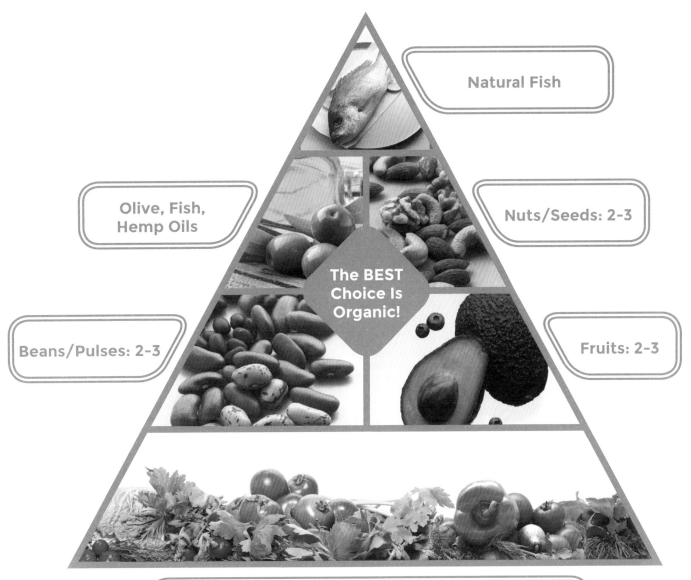

Natural Fish

Olive, Fish, Hemp Oils

Nuts/Seeds: 2-3

The BEST Choice Is Organic!

Beans/Pulses: 2-3

Fruits: 2-3

**Vegetables (excluding root): 8-12 servings a day
1/2 raw veggies: Salads, etc.**

7. Stay Active Daily.

Contrary to the opinion of fitness fanatics, there are two simple ways to get your body working better and stronger. And no, they do not include swimming and cycling, although you can add these later if you want to.

One of the two simple ways to exercise is to build up to walking 3-5 miles per day, in a fast, purposely strong way with as long a stride as you can. Keep your hands moving from chest level to belt level as you move with each stride.

Use weights or wrist weights as you improve.

If this is difficult for you at the start, and your lungs are weak, then lie down to exercise to make it easier.

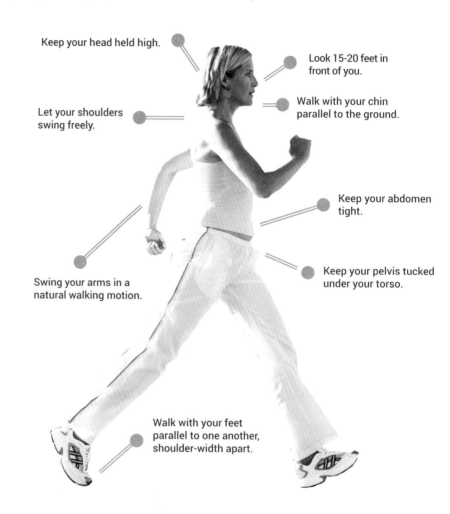

Keep your head held high.

Look 15-20 feet in front of you.

Walk with your chin parallel to the ground.

Let your shoulders swing freely.

Keep your abdomen tight.

Keep your pelvis tucked under your torso.

Swing your arms in a natural walking motion.

Walk with your feet parallel to one another, shoulder-width apart.

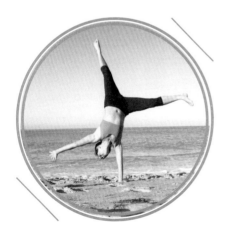

Lie down in a comfortable place. On your bed (if it's firm enough), when you first wake up is a great time and place for this. Bring a knee up to your chest as high as you can get it and then alternate with the other knee. Do as many of these as you can while keeping count. Do this every day and set yourself targets to increase the speed and the number as the weeks go by. You should be doing enough to make your lungs and heart beat faster. At the same time, as you improve your count on your back you need to be starting your walking and building this up.

The second great exercise for strengthening your lungs is to build up slowly where you can exercise at maximum rate for 2 minutes, 6 times per day. It does not matter what exercise you do, e.g. skipping, star jumps, running on the spot; just about anything, as long as your heart and lungs are working at maximum capacity. By working at maximum rate, your lungs and muscles connected with your heart and lungs will get stronger, and health will balance perfectly.

Physical activity is vital to your rehabilitation plan.

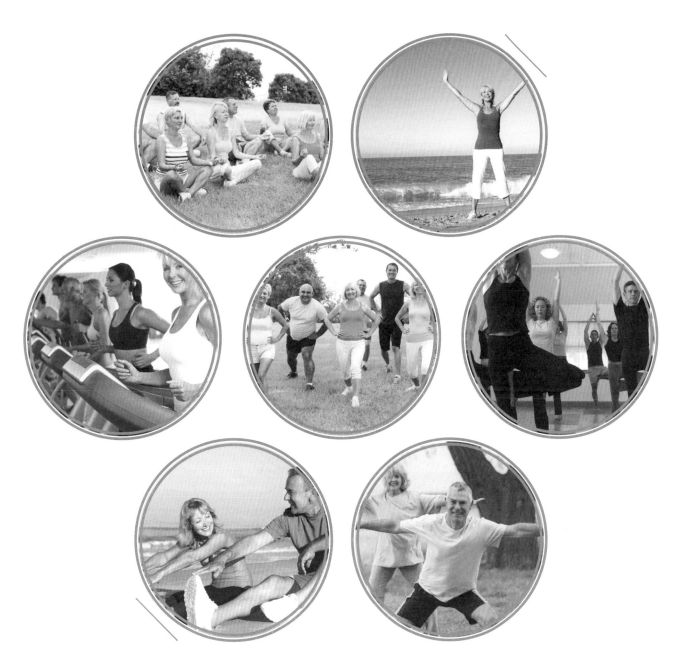

8. Learn Proper Breathing.

> *Breathing properly is critical since oxygen is the foundation of overall health.*

There are two types of breathing:

1. **Anxious Breathing:** In the chest.

2. **Relaxed Breathing:** In the diaphragm or stomach area.

The first type of breathing in the chest is related to a stress response and includes hormones like cortisol. This stressful breathing should only be temporary since it is related to a fight-or-flight response that causes hormones to release to relax breathing. If stressful breathing grows chronic, the body will retain carbon dioxide and cortisol to affect healthy functioning systems. Stress breathing will also cause the immune system to weaken, leaving it susceptible to infection.

Make it your number one goal to retrain your body to breathe in a relaxed, healthy manner. This will clear out carbon dioxide and cortisol. When carbon dioxide builds up in your bloodstream, it will destroy a substance called hemoglobin that the blood uses to transport oxygen throughout the body. This is why it's especially important to focus on relaxed breathing that comes from the diaphragm.

How to Breathe Correctly

The easiest way to relearn correct breathing is to lie flat on your back on the floor, on a mat or blanket or on a firm bed. Place a small weighted object on your belly button, like a heavy book. Take a deep breath in through your nose so that the book rises as your stomach, or diaphragm, fills with air. Hold this deep breath for a count of 4 and then release through your nose so that your stomach deflates. Use this process to release any tension as you exhale

and repeat. In the exercise, your chest should not move to indicate relaxed, stress-free breathing.

Practice this low-stress breathing exercise again and again as you lie down. Once you have mastered the rhythm of the calming breath, you can start to try the exercise while standing. Initially, you may feel dizzy as you intake more and more fresh oxygen, but it's still important to practice the exercise whenever you can.

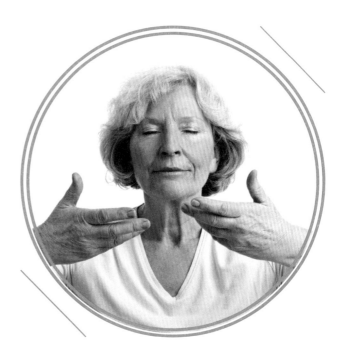

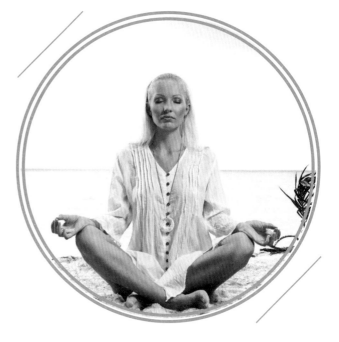

9. Stimulate Acupressure Points.

Another component in your Rehabilitation Plan is to stimulate acupressure points that connect to your kidney health recovery system. There are a number of points that can be massaged gently with a finger to mimic actual acupuncture. Please read more about this on **page 37**.

10. Get More Sun Exposure.

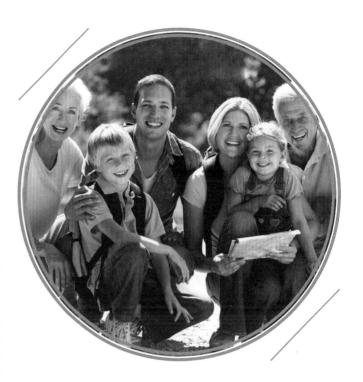

An essential vitamin to support your overall health is vitamin D3. You can find a large dose of vitamin D3 in the recommended supplement on **page 35**, but it's still critical to get some natural vitamin D from sun exposure.

The sun is the source of life. Unfortunately, myths have been circulated in the health community that the sun is an enemy that we must stay away from at all costs. Even worse, many health professionals recommend slathering your body in toxic chemicals every time you go out in the sun. Of course, I'm not recommending lying in the sun for 6 hours at once on the first hot day of the year. It's essential to build up the skin's tolerance to sun exposure over several weeks for natural protection. By the time that hot summer days come around, you will be able to tolerate a greater amount of natural sun exposure.

Recommendations for sun exposure:

- **Expose as much skin as you can to the sun each day, such as on your morning walk.**

- **Build up your sun exposure gradually from spring to summer seasons.**

- **Try to stay out of the sun in mid-day without a cover-up; a cover-up is preferred to sunscreen.**

- **If you do use sunscreen or sun cream, purchase organic products instead of chemical-based, name-brand creams.**

- **It's important to remember that the sun is your friend, and sunshine can be enjoyed in moderation!**

More About Clearing Inflammation and Promoting Healing

Nascent Iodine Colloidal Drops

Nascent Iodine is Iodine in its atomic form, rather than its molecular form. Nascent Iodine is a totally different form of Iodine from its denser state where it is sold as an antiseptic. All the cells in your body contain and make use of Iodine. It is concentrated in the glandular system of the body, with your thyroid containing the highest amount compared to any other organ.

Nascent Iodine supports the thyroid and the immune system, as well as regulating the metabolism.

> **Ingredients:**
>
> • Iodine (in its atomic form) – 400mcg

Dosage:
Take 5 drops, 3 times per day in 20ml of water, swish around the mouth for 30 seconds before swallowing. Build over 2 weeks to 15 x 3 until well and then slowly reduce back to 5 x 3. Take 1st dose on waking, 2nd mid-morning, and 3rd mid-afternoon.

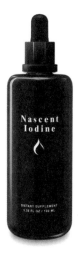

BlockBuster AllClear™

BlockBuster AllClear™ is, by any measure, the best and most powerful enzyme formula available. This carefully formulated blend of powerful enzymes such as Serrapeptase, Nattokinase, Digestive Enzyme, antioxidants, and proanthocyanidins (including Grape Seed Extract and Pycnogenol) is now in a delayed release capsule – all with a long history of studies and a reputation for great effect.

BlockBuster contains Serrapeptase to provide powerful support for the digestive system and lower inflammation. BlockBuster is perfect for those requiring the highest level of support for their health or long-term maintenance.

> **Ingredients:**
>
> • Serrapeptase - 80,000 IU
> • Nattokinase* - 1600 FU
> • Protease - 20,000 HUT
> • Lipase - 1500 FIP
> • Amylase - 4000 DU
> • Cellulase - 600 CU
> • Lactase - 1000 ALU
> • Acerola extract - 50 mg
> • Amla extract - 50 mg
> • Olive Leaf Citrus Blend - 230 mg
> • Trace Minerals (Coral Calcium) - 100 mg
> • Bacillus Coagulans - 376,000,000 CFU
> • Protease S - 5 mg
> • Grapeseed extract - 100 mg
> • Policosanol - 6 mg
> • Pycnogenol® - 10 mg

Dosage:
Take 2 capsules, 3 times per day, 30 minutes before eating a meal with water; reduce to 1 x 3 after a month.

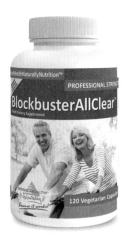

More About Missing Nutrients

Curcuminx4000

Curcuminx4000 provides superior support and pain relief for digestive problems, the liver, and the gallbladder. Curcumin also has well-established properties that compare to supplemental vitamins C and E in their antioxidant abilities to neutralize free radicals.

Ingredients:

- Meriva ® (root) Curcuma longa extract - 600mg

Dosage:

Take 1 capsule, 3 times per day with the BlockBuster.

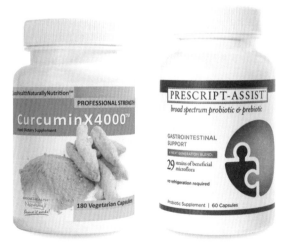

Prescript-Assist - 29 Super Strain Probiotic

Prescript-Assist is the next-generation, clinically-proven vegan probiotic supplement. It maintains healthy GI tract microfloral ecologies, supports the gut immune system, and promotes normal bowel function.

Ingredients:

Each 600mg capsule of Prescript-Assist contains a proprietary blend of Leonardite and the following Class I beneficial microorganisms:

- *Anthrobacteragilis, Anthrobactercitreus, Anthrobacterglobiformis, Anthrobacterluteus, Anthrobacter simplex, Acinetobactercalcoaceticus, Aztobacterchroococcum, Azotobacterpaspali, Azospirillumbrasiliense, Azospirillumlipoferum, Bacillus polymyxa, Bacillus subtilis, Bacteroideslipolyticum, Bacteriodessuccinogenes, Brevibacteriumlipolyticum, Brevibacteriumstationis, Kurthazopfil, Myrotheciumverrucaria, Pseudomonas calcis, Pseudomonas dentrificans, Pseudomonas flourescens, Pseudomonas glathei, Phanerochaetechrysoporium, Streptomyces fradiae, Streptomyces celluslosae, Streptomyces griseoflavus*

Other ingredients:

- Cellulose (vegetarian capsule)

Dosage:

Take 1 capsule, 2 times a day; can be opened and mixed with food. Then take for maintenance at the rate of 1 every 3 days.

B4 Health Spray

B4 Health Spray may support healthy homocysteine levels, the heart and cardiovascular system, proper vitamin B12 absorption through the digestive tract, and a healthy immune system.

Ingredients:

- Vitamin C (as ascorbic acid) - 60mg
- Vitamin D (as cholecalciferol) - 400IU
- Vitamin E (as D-alpha tocopherol acetate) - 30IU
- Thiamin (Vitamin B1) as (Thiamin HCL) - 1.5mg
- Riboflavin (Vitamin B2) (as Riboflavin) - 1.7mg
- Niacin (Vitamin B3) (Niacinamide) - 20mg
- Vitamin B6 (as Pyridoxine HCL) - 2mg
- Folate (as Folic Acid) - 400mcg
- Vitamin B12 (as Methylcobalamin) - 6mcg
- Biotin - 300mcg
- Pantothenic Acid (Vitamin B5) (as D-Calcium Pantothenate) - 10mg
- Magnesium (as Magnesium gluconate) - 400mcg
- Selenium (as Selebium amino acid) - 70mcg
- Proprietary Complex - Trimethylglycine, N-Acetyl-D-Glucosamine, Ribose, Taurine, Grapeseed Extract, Pine Bark Extract, Co-Enzyme Q10 - 63mg

Other Ingredients:

De-ionized water, glycerin, aloe vera extract, trace minerals, stevia (leaf), grapefruit seed extract, potassium sorbate, natural flavors.

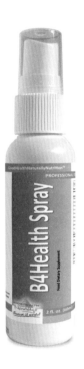

Dosage:
Take 6 sprays daily.

More About Immune Strengthening Formulations

D.I.P. Daily Immune Protection™

D.I.P. Daily Immune Protection™ is designed to support the fight against infection, boost the immune response to allergens, strengthen healthy cells, and balance the immune system.

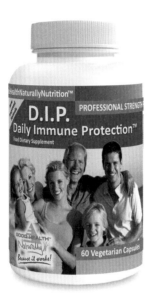

Ingredients:

- Vitamin C (from Ascorbic Acid) – 120mg
- Vitamin D3 (from Cholecalciferol) – 1000IU
- ExSelen (2% Selenium) – 100mcg
- Zinc Glycinate Chelate 20%
- Epicor (dried yeast fermentate) – 500mg
- Dimethylglycine HCL – 250mg
- Elderberry Fruit Extract 4:1 – 200mg
- Larch Arabinogalactan Powder – 200mg
- Immune Assist – Micron Powder – 80mg
- Beta Glucan 1,3 (Glucan 85%) – 60mg

Other ingredients:

- Vegetable cellulose (capsule), medium chain triglycerides, and rice bran.

Dosage:
Take 1 capsule, twice daily with food.

Kidney Rescue

Kidney Rescue cleanses the liver, while providing adrenal support. Kidney Rescue may also support the lymphatic system (lungs, kidneys, liver, colon, and skin), adrenal glands, ligaments, and joints.

Ingredients:

Proprietary Blend: 1455 mg
- Cinnamon Bark
- Cedar Leaves
- Lycci Fructus
- Wild Rose Root
- Fenugreek Seed
- Holy Basil Powder
- Borage Leaves
- Damiana Leaf
- Red Raspberry Leaf
- Cloves Powder
- Pygeum Bark
- Cayenne

Other Ingredients:

Croscarmellose sodium, dicalcium phosphate dihydrate, silicon dioxide, magnesium stearate, stearic acid

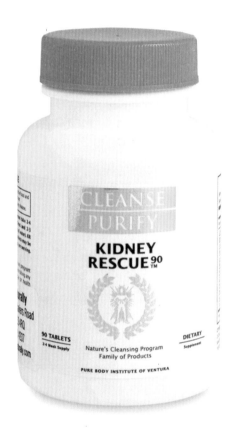

Dosage:
Take 2-5 tablets, 5 times per day, 6 days per week.

More About Optional Nutrients

Ultimate Immune System Support Kit – 1st Line (Thiocyanate) Immune Support Kit

Sodium Thiocyanate and Sodium Hypothiocyanate can provide strong immunity against the first signs of infection. 1st Line clears any infections that may reside in the cells and provides a strong defense against viruses, yeasts, and fungi.

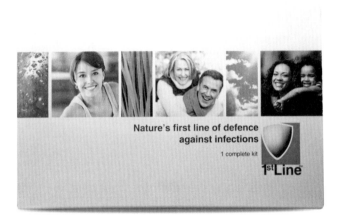

Nature's first line of defence against infections
1 complete kit
1st Line

Ingredients:

- Sodium Thiocyanate – 100ppm
- Sodium Hypothiocyanate – 60ppm

Dosage:

Take 1 kit daily for 3 days (total of 3). 1st Line should always be taken at least 90 minutes before and after food, approximately. 3 kits are the minimum, and in serious conditions, 10 kits over 10 days are better if finances allow.

More About Acupuncture

Stimulating the points in page 1.23 of the book **Mastering Acupuncture** will help to balance kidney health. These points can be effectively and safely stimulated using the **HealthPoint™** electro-acupressure kit. The advantage of the kit is it gives you the power to precisely locate the acupuncture point, and indeed other points, so you can enjoy the benefits of acupuncture at home and without any needles.

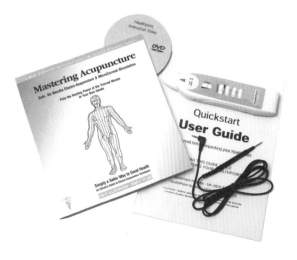

HealthPoint™ is easy to use, painless, and effective. It includes an instructional DVD and book covering over 150 pain and non-pain conditions that can be helped, such as headaches, back, neck, and joint problems.

The gentle and systematic stimulation of the body's natural healing system can speed recovery in many cases. **HealthPoint™** breakthrough technology was developed by leading pain control specialist Dr. Julian Kenyon, MD 21 years ago, and today features the latest microchip technology to quickly locate acupuncture points key to specific health conditions, such as the points for chronic kidney disease.

In Conclusion:

The Kidney Rehabilitation Program offers a complete rehabilitation plan that is specially designed to comprehensively prevent or manage your kidney disease.

Kidney disease can better be understood as a lifestyle disease. This means that if you change your lifestyle, there is a great chance of partial or full recovery. When you implement the changes found in the 10 Step Plan, your body can naturally begin the healing process to recover your health.

❧ *Drugs won't improve your health.*

Drugs aren't effective since they can't make you healthy again. In a best-case scenario, drugs may provide some relief. In a worst-case scenario, they will further damage your health and can even cause untimely death.

Of course, the pharmaceutical industry would love you to continue on your current drug regimen and ineffective rehabilitation plan, relying on toxic medications that inhibit your true path to long-term healing.

❧ *Thankfully, you have discovered that there is a better way*

You can use the Kidney Rehabilitation Program to prevent or manage kidney disease, even if other medical alternatives have not worked for you:

- **This program will help you to embrace your health and improve your quality of life in a rehabilitation plan that includes education, coaching, and exercise.**

- **This program will incorporate support and therapy to provide assistance so that you can achieve the best results possible.**

You will find the Kidney Rehabilitation Program outlined in this book. When you follow it carefully, you will see some results starting within weeks.

❧ *This rehabilitation plan will always offer health improvements.*

The worst outcome when using this plan will be that your health improves, but you still need to take some drugs if your health has been damaged irreparably by medication or kidney disease.

❧ *Start slowly and begin rehabilitation step-by-step.*

If you're not used to making major changes in your life, it may be difficult to adopt new healthy habits at first. But stick with it because...

❧ *Your health is invaluable...*

Robert Redfern, Your Health Coach

Email: robert@goodhealth.nu
www.MyGoodHealthClub.com
for step by step coaching and support.

Daily Kidney Rehabilitation Plan

TIME	ACTION	AMOUNT
Just before eating	1st Line Kit	Take 1 kit daily for 3 days; should be taken 90 minutes before and 90 minutes after food, approximately

BREAKFAST

TIME	ACTION	AMOUNT
30 minutes before breakfast	Nascent Iodine Drops	Take 5 drops in 20ml of water, swish around the mouth for 30 seconds before swallowing
30 minutes before breakfast	BlockBuster AllClear	Take 2 capsules before eating with water
With breakfast	Curcuminx4000	Take 1 capsule with the BlockBuster
With breakfast	Kidney Rescue	Take 2 tablets
With breakfast	Prescript-Assist	Take 1 capsule
With breakfast	D.I.P.	Take 1 capsule

BREAK

TIME	ACTION	AMOUNT
Break	Kidney Rescue	Take 2 tablets

LUNCH

TIME	ACTION	AMOUNT
30 minutes before lunch	Nascent Iodine Drops	Take 5 drops in 20ml of water, swish around the mouth for 30 seconds before swallowing
30 minutes before lunch	BlockBuster AllClear	Take 2 capsules before eating with water
With lunch	Curcuminx4000	Take 1 capsule with the BlockBuster
With lunch	B4 Health Spray	Take 6 sprays in the mouth
With lunch	Kidney Rescue	Take 2 tablets

BREAK

TIME	ACTION	AMOUNT
Break	Kidney Rescue	Take 2 tablets

DINNER

TIME	ACTION	AMOUNT
30 minutes before diner	Nascent Iodine Drops	Take 5 drops in 20ml of water, swish around the mouth for 30 seconds before swallowing
30 minutes before dinner	BlockBuster AllClear	Take 2 capsules before eating with water
With dinner	Curcuminx4000	Take 1 capsule with the BlockBuster
With dinner	Kidney Rescue	Take 2 tablets
With dinner	Prescript-Assist	Take 1 capsule
With dinner	D.I.P.	Take 1 capsule

All the books in this series:

- **Diabetes**
- **Liver Health**
- **Digestive Problems**
- **Colitis**
- **Crohn's Disease**
- **IBS**
- **Gallbladder**
- **Constipation**
- **Thyroid Health**

Other Books by Robert Redfern:

- **The 'Miracle Enzyme' Is Serrapeptase**
- **Turning A Blind Eye**
- **Mastering Acupuncture**
- **EquiHealth Equine Acupressure**